This 21 Day Bulletproof Keto Diet Workbook Belongs to:

_____

ISBN: 9781070519524

**Day 1
Starting Weight
and
Measurements**

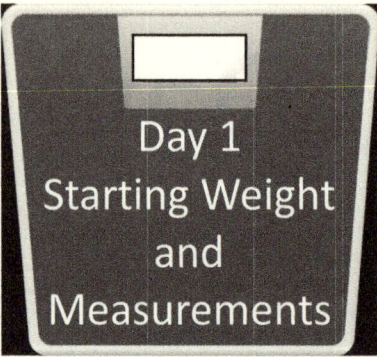

I Can and I Will!

Target Weight ⟶ _____

Starting Measurements:

Right Bicep _____

Left Bicep _____

Chest _____

Waist _____

Hips _____

Right Thigh _____

Left Thigh _____

Right Calf _____

Left Calf _____

Before

4"x6"

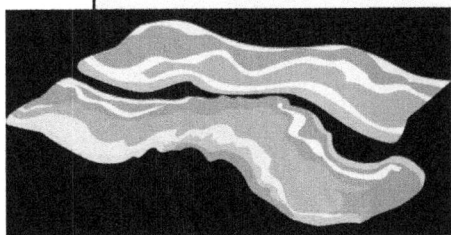
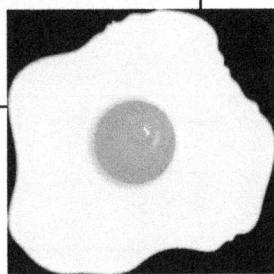

Questions To Ask Myself

Why am I starting the Keto lifestyle?

_____

_____

_____

_____

What's my end goal?

_____

_____

_____

_____

Do I have a weight loss mindset?

_____

_____

_____

_____

Who can I count on for support?

_____

_____

_____

_____

Day 1 - 7

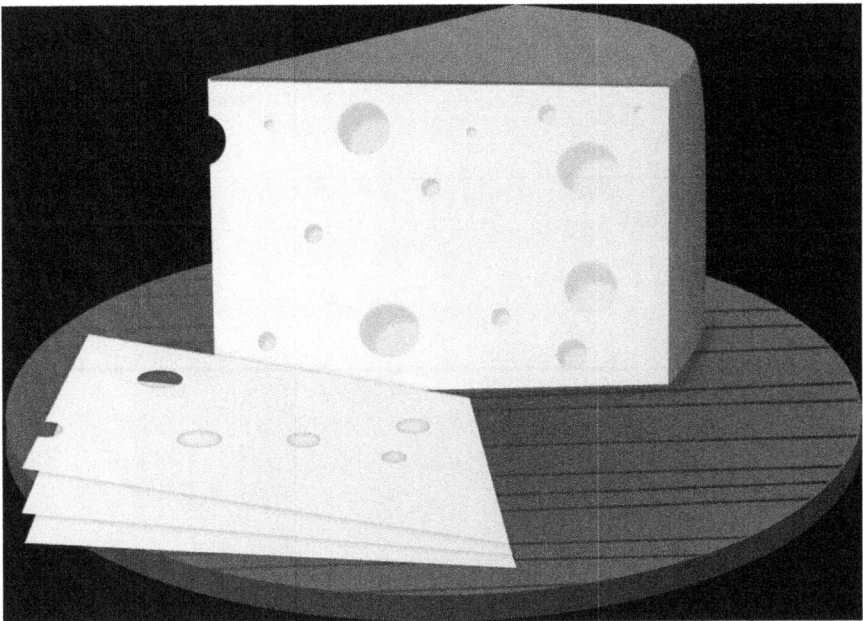

Meal Planner   Day 1 - 7

Day 1	Breakfast: Lunch: Dinner:
Day 2	Breakfast: Lunch: Dinner:
Day 3	Breakfast: Lunch: Dinner:
Day 4	Breakfast: Lunch: Dinner:
Day 5	Breakfast: Lunch: Dinner:
Day 6	Breakfast: Lunch: Dinner:
Day 7	Breakfast: Lunch: Dinner:
Snacks	

Shopping   Day 1 - 7

MEAT & FISH	DAIRY	VEGETABLES
Bacon	Heavy Cream	Broccoli
Ground Beef	Full Fat Yogurt	Cauliflower
Chicken	Eggs	Cabbage
Cold Cuts	Butter	Cucumber
Pork	Ghee	Eggplant
Lamb	Sour Cream	Bell Pepper
Organ Meats	Cream Cheese	Asparagus
Duck	Full Fat Cheeses	Salad Mix
Steak	**PANTRY**	Spaghetti Squash
Sausage	Pork Rinds	Zuchinni
Shrimp	Almond Milk	Onions
Salmon	Coconut Milk	Garlic
Tuna	Coffee	Celery
FATS & OILS	Himalayan Pink Salt	**FRUITS**
Olive Oil	Mustard	Avocados
Avocado Oil	90% Dark Chocolate	Blueberries
Sesame Oil	Almond Flour	Blackberries
MCT Oil	Coconut Flour	Raspberries
Lard	Bone Broth	Strawberries
Cocoa Butter	Xanthan Gum	Lemons
Coconut Oil	Erythritol	Limes
Nut Butters	Monkfruit	Nuts & Seeds

Shopping List

Day 1 - 7

MEAT & FISH	DAIRY	VEGETABLES
	PANTRY	

FATS & OILS		FRUITS

Habit Tracker

HABIT	1	2	3	4	5	6	7	REWARD

Mood

DAY	MOOD					WHY?
1	☺	☺	☹	☹	☹	
2	☺	☺	☹	☹	☹	
3	☺	☺	☹	☹	☹	
4	☺	☺	☹	☹	☹	
5	☺	☺	☹	☹	☹	
6	☺	☺	☹	☹	☹	
7	☺	☺	☹	☹	☹	

Only I can change my life. No one can do it for me.

Exercise Tracker   Day 1 - 7

Day 1	Day 2	Day 3
Cardio ○ Weights ○	Cardio ○ Weights ○	Cardio ○ Weights ○

Day 4	Day 5	Day 6
Cardio ○ Weights ○	Cardio ○ Weights ○	Cardio ○ Weights ○

Day 7	Day	Calories Burned
	1	
	2	
	3	
	4	
	5	
Cardio ○	6	
Weights ○	7	

Day 1 Food Tracker

Date: _____

MON TUE WED THU FRI SAT SUN

⊕ Daily Target						

Breakfast	Calories	Fat	Protein	Carbs	Fiber	Net Carbs
Total:						

Lunch	Calories	Fat	Protein	Carbs	Fiber	Net Carbs
Total:						

Dinner	Calories	Fat	Protein	Carbs	Fiber	Net Carbs
Total:						

Snacks	Calories	Fat	Protein	Carbs	Fiber	Net Carbs
Total:						

Daily Total						

Ketosis: Y/N   Intermittent Fasting: From _____am/pm - To_____am/pm

How'd I do?

Day 2 Food Tracker

Date: _____
MON TUE WED THU FRI SAT SUN

Daily Target						

Breakfast	Calories	Fat	Protein	Carbs	Fiber	Net Carbs
Total:						

Lunch	Calories	Fat	Protein	Carbs	Fiber	Net Carbs
Total:						

Dinner	Calories	Fat	Protein	Carbs	Fiber	Net Carbs
Total:						

Snacks	Calories	Fat	Protein	Carbs	Fiber	Net Carbs
Total:						

Daily Total						

Ketosis: Y/N   Intermittent Fasting: From _____am/pm - To_____am/pm

How'd I do?

Day 3 Food Tracker

⊕ Daily Target						
Breakfast	Calories	Fat	Protein	Carbs	Fiber	Net Carbs
Total:						
Lunch	Calories	Fat	Protein	Carbs	Fiber	Net Carbs
Total:						
Dinner	Calories	Fat	Protein	Carbs	Fiber	Net Carbs
Total:						
Snacks	Calories	Fat	Protein	Carbs	Fiber	Net Carbs
Total:						
Daily Total						

Ketosis: Y/N   Intermittent Fasting: From _____am/pm - To_____am/pm

How'd I do?

Day 4 Food Tracker

Date: _____
MON TUE WED THU FRI SAT SUN

Daily Target						
Breakfast	Calories	Fat	Protein	Carbs	Fiber	Net Carbs
Total:						
Lunch	Calories	Fat	Protein	Carbs	Fiber	Net Carbs
Total:						
Dinner	Calories	Fat	Protein	Carbs	Fiber	Net Carbs
Total:						
Snacks	Calories	Fat	Protein	Carbs	Fiber	Net Carbs
Total:						
Daily Total						

Ketosis: Y/N   Intermittent Fasting: From _____am/pm - To_____am/pm

How'd I do?

Day 5 Food Tracker

Date: _____

MON TUE WED THU FRI SAT SUN

🎯 Daily Target						

Breakfast	Calories	Fat	Protein	Carbs	Fiber	Net Carbs
Total:						

Lunch	Calories	Fat	Protein	Carbs	Fiber	Net Carbs
Total:						

Dinner	Calories	Fat	Protein	Carbs	Fiber	Net Carbs
Total:						

Snacks	Calories	Fat	Protein	Carbs	Fiber	Net Carbs
Total:						

Daily Total						

Ketosis: Y/N   Intermittent Fasting: From _____am/pm - To_____am/pm

How'd I do?

Day 6 Food Tracker

Date: _____

MON TUE WED THU FRI SAT SUN

🎯 Daily Target						

Breakfast	Calories	Fat	Protein	Carbs	Fiber	Net Carbs
Total:						

Lunch	Calories	Fat	Protein	Carbs	Fiber	Net Carbs
Total:						

Dinner	Calories	Fat	Protein	Carbs	Fiber	Net Carbs
Total:						

Snacks	Calories	Fat	Protein	Carbs	Fiber	Net Carbs
Total:						

Daily Total						

Ketosis: Y/N   Intermittent Fasting: From _____am/pm - To_____am/pm

How'd I do?

_____
_____
_____
_____
_____
_____
_____
_____
_____
_____
_____
_____
_____
_____
_____
_____
_____
_____
_____

Day 7 Food Tracker

⊕ Daily Target						
Breakfast	Calories	Fat	Protein	Carbs	Fiber	Net Carbs
Total:						
Lunch	Calories	Fat	Protein	Carbs	Fiber	Net Carbs
Total:						
Dinner	Calories	Fat	Protein	Carbs	Fiber	Net Carbs
Total:						
Snacks	Calories	Fat	Protein	Carbs	Fiber	Net Carbs
Total:						
Daily Total						

Ketosis: Y/N   Intermittent Fasting: From _____am/pm - To_____am/pm

How'd I do?

| Day 8 Starting Weight and Measurements | Slow and Steady Wins the Race! |

Weight +/- ⟹ _____

Measurements After 7 Days:

Right Bicep _____

Left Bicep _____

Chest _____

Waist _____

Hips _____

Right Thigh _____

Left Thigh _____

Right Calf _____

Left Calf _____

After 7 Days

4"x6"

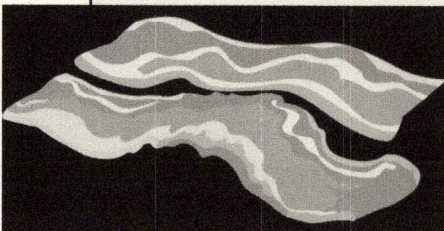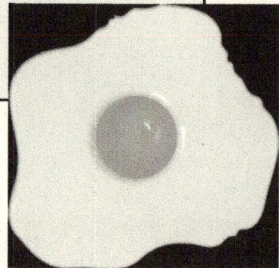

Questions To Ask Yourself

Am I happy with how I did my first 7 days?

_____

_____

_____

_____

What was my biggest win?

_____

_____

_____

What can I do better at?

_____

_____

_____

How does my body feel?

_____

_____

_____

Day 8 - 14

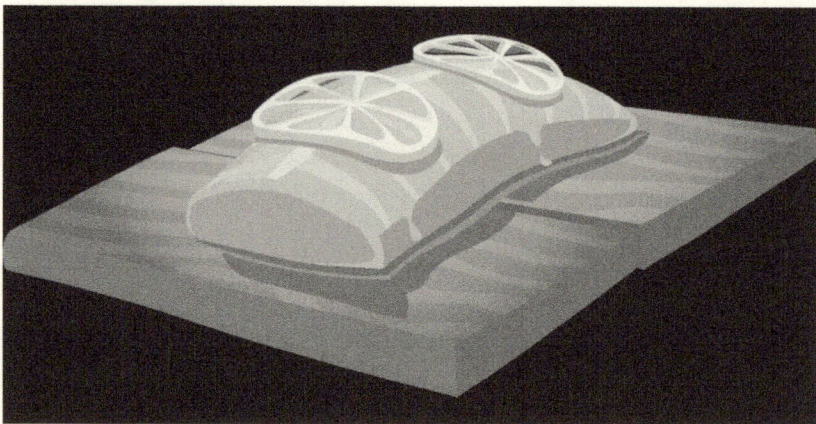

Meal Planner

Day 8 - 14

Day 8	Breakfast: Lunch: Dinner:
Day 9	Breakfast: Lunch: Dinner:
Day 10	Breakfast: Lunch: Dinner:
Day 11	Breakfast: Lunch: Dinner:
Day 12	Breakfast: Lunch: Dinner:
Day 13	Breakfast: Lunch: Dinner:
Day 14	Breakfast: Lunch: Dinner:
Snacks	

Shopping List   Day 8-14

MEAT & FISH	DAIRY	VEGETABLES
Bacon	Heavy Cream	Broccoli
Ground Beef	Full Fat Yogurt	Cauliflower
Chicken	Eggs	Cabbage
Cold Cuts	Butter	Cucumber
Pork	Ghee	Eggplant
Lamb	Sour Cream	Bell Pepper
Organ Meats	Cream Cheese	Asparagus
Duck	Full Fat Cheeses	Salad Mix
Steak	**PANTRY**	Spaghetti Squash
Sausage	Pork Rinds	Zucchini
Shrimp	Almond Milk	Onions
Salmon	Coconut Milk	Garlic
Tuna	Coffee	Celery
FATS & OILS	Himalayan Pink Salt	**FRUITS**
Olive Oil	Mustard	Avocados
Avocado Oil	90% Dark Chocolate	Blueberries
Sesame Oil	Almond Flour	Blackberries
MCT Oil	Coconut Flour	Raspberries
Lard	Bone Broth	Strawberries
Cocoa Butter	Xanthan Gum	Lemons
Coconut Oil	Erythritol	Limes
Nut Butters	Monkfruit	Nuts & Seeds

Shopping List　　　　Day 8 - 14

MEAT & FISH	DAIRY	VEGETABLES
	PANTRY	
FATS & OILS		**FRUITS**

Habit Tracker

HABIT	8	9	10	11	12	13	14	REWARD

Mood

DAY	MOOD					WHY?
8	☺	☺	☹	☹	☹	
9	☺	☺	☹	☹	☹	
10	☺	☺	☹	☹	☹	
11	☺	☺	☹	☹	☹	
12	☺	☺	☹	☹	☹	
13	☺	☺	☹	☹	☹	
14	☺	☺	☹	☹	☹	

If you are tired of starting over Stop giving up!

Exercise Tracker Day 8 - 14

Day 8	Day 9	Day 10
Cardio ○ Weights ○	Cardio ○ Weights ○	Cardio ○ Weights ○

Day 11	Day 12	Day 13
Cardio ○ Weights ○	Cardio ○ Weights ○	Cardio ○ Weights ○

Day 14	Day	Calories Burned
	8	
	9	
	10	
	11	
	12	
Cardio ○ Weights ○	13	
	14	

Day 8 Food Tracker

🎯 Daily Target						
Breakfast	Calories	Fat	Protein	Carbs	Fiber	Net Carbs
Total:						
Lunch	Calories	Fat	Protein	Carbs	Fiber	Net Carbs
Total:						
Dinner	Calories	Fat	Protein	Carbs	Fiber	Net Carbs
Total:						
Snacks	Calories	Fat	Protein	Carbs	Fiber	Net Carbs
Total:						
Daily Total						

Ketosis: Y/N   Intermittent Fasting: From _____am/pm - To_____am/pm

How'd I do?

Day 9 Food Tracker

Date: _____
MON TUE WED THU FRI SAT SUN

⊕ Daily Target						
Breakfast	Calories	Fat	Protein	Carbs	Fiber	Net Carbs
Total:						
Lunch	Calories	Fat	Protein	Carbs	Fiber	Net Carbs
Total:						
Dinner	Calories	Fat	Protein	Carbs	Fiber	Net Carbs
Total:						
Snacks	Calories	Fat	Protein	Carbs	Fiber	Net Carbs
Total:						
Daily Total						

Ketosis: Y/N   Intermittent Fasting: From _____am/pm - To_____am/pm

How'd I do?

Day 10 Food Tracker

⊕ Daily Target						
Breakfast	Calories	Fat	Protein	Carbs	Fiber	Net Carbs
Total:						
Lunch	Calories	Fat	Protein	Carbs	Fiber	Net Carbs
Total:						
Dinner	Calories	Fat	Protein	Carbs	Fiber	Net Carbs
Total:						
Snacks	Calories	Fat	Protein	Carbs	Fiber	Net Carbs
Total:						
Daily Total						

Ketosis: Y/N   Intermittent Fasting: From _____am/pm - To_____am/pm

How'd I do?

Day 11 Food Tracker

Date: _____

MON TUE WED THU FRI SAT SUN

🎯 Daily Target						
Breakfast	Calories	Fat	Protein	Carbs	Fiber	Net Carbs
Total:						
Lunch	Calories	Fat	Protein	Carbs	Fiber	Net Carbs
Total:						
Dinner	Calories	Fat	Protein	Carbs	Fiber	Net Carbs
Total:						
Snacks	Calories	Fat	Protein	Carbs	Fiber	Net Carbs
Total:						
Daily Total						

Ketosis: Y/N   Intermittent Fasting: From _____am/pm - To_____am/pm

How'd I do?

Day 12 Food Tracker

⊕ Daily Target						
Breakfast	Calories	Fat	Protein	Carbs	Fiber	Net Carbs
Total:						
Lunch	Calories	Fat	Protein	Carbs	Fiber	Net Carbs
Total:						
Dinner	Calories	Fat	Protein	Carbs	Fiber	Net Carbs
Total:						
Snacks	Calories	Fat	Protein	Carbs	Fiber	Net Carbs
Total:						
Daily Total						

Ketosis: Y/N   Intermittent Fasting: From _____am/pm - To_____am/pm

How'd I do?

Day 13 Food Tracker

Date: _____

MON TUE WED THU FRI SAT SUN

🎯 Daily Target						
Breakfast	Calories	Fat	Protein	Carbs	Fiber	Net Carbs
Total:						
Lunch	Calories	Fat	Protein	Carbs	Fiber	Net Carbs
Total:						
Dinner	Calories	Fat	Protein	Carbs	Fiber	Net Carbs
Total:						
Snacks	Calories	Fat	Protein	Carbs	Fiber	Net Carbs
Total:						
Daily Total						

Ketosis: Y/N   Intermittent Fasting: From _____am/pm - To_____am/pm

How'd I do?

Day 14 Food Tracker

Date: _____
MON TUE WED THU FRI SAT SUN

⊕ Daily Target						
Breakfast	Calories	Fat	Protein	Carbs	Fiber	Net Carbs
Total:						
Lunch	Calories	Fat	Protein	Carbs	Fiber	Net Carbs
Total:						
Dinner	Calories	Fat	Protein	Carbs	Fiber	Net Carbs
Total:						
Snacks	Calories	Fat	Protein	Carbs	Fiber	Net Carbs
Total:						
Daily Total						

Ketosis: Y/N   Intermittent Fasting: From _____am/pm - To_____am/pm

How'd I do?

Day 15
Starting Weight
and
Measurements

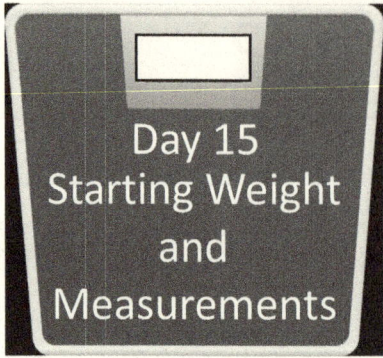

Be stronger than your excuses

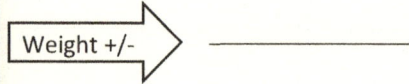

Weight +/- ⟶ _____

Measurements After 14 Days:

Right Bicep _____

Left Bicep _____

Chest _____

Waist _____

Hips _____

Right Thigh _____

Left Thigh _____

Right Calf _____

Left Calf _____

After 14 Days

4"x6"

Questions To Ask Yourself

Is it getting easier or harder to stick to Keto? Why?

_____

_____

_____

_____

What's my biggest issue with eating the Keto way?

_____

_____

_____

_____

Is there anything I can do to make it easier?

_____

_____

_____

_____

What is the food I miss most? Is there a Keto substitute for it?

_____

_____

_____

_____

Day 15 - 21

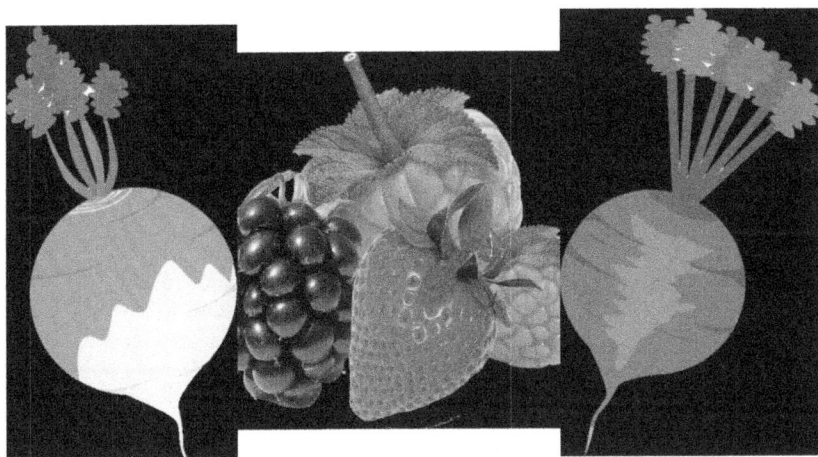

Meal Planner

Day 15 - 21

Day 15	Breakfast: Lunch: Dinner:
Day 16	Breakfast: Lunch: Dinner:
Day 17	Breakfast: Lunch: Dinner:
Day 18	Breakfast: Lunch: Dinner:
Day 19	Breakfast: Lunch: Dinner:
Day 20	Breakfast: Lunch: Dinner:
Day 21	Breakfast: Lunch: Dinner:
Snacks	

Shopping List   Day 15 - 21

MEAT & FISH	DAIRY	VEGETABLES
Bacon	Heavy Cream	Broccoli
Ground Beef	Full Fat Yogurt	Cauliflower
Chicken	Eggs	Cabbage
Cold Cuts	Butter	Cucumber
Pork	Ghee	Eggplant
Lamb	Sour Cream	Bell Pepper
Organ Meats	Cream Cheese	Asparagus
Duck	Full Fat Cheeses	Salad Mix
Steak	**PANTRY**	Spaghetti Squash
Sausage	Pork Rinds	Zucchini
Shrimp	Almond Milk	Onions
Salmon	Coconut Milk	Garlic
Tuna	Coffee	Celery
FATS & OILS	Himalayan Pink Salt	**FRUITS**
Olive Oil	Mustard	Avocados
Avocado Oil	90% Dark Chocolate	Blueberries
Sesame Oil	Almond Flour	Blackberries
MCT Oil	Coconut Flour	Raspberries
Lard	Bone Broth	Strawberries
Cocoa Butter	Xanthan Gum	Lemons
Coconut Oil	Erythritol	Limes
Nut Butters	Monkfruit	Nuts & Seeds

Shopping List   Day 15 -21

MEAT & FISH	DAIRY	VEGETABLES
	PANTRY	

FATS & OILS		FRUITS

Habit Tracker

HABIT	15	16	17	18	19	20	21	REWARD

Mood

DAY	MOOD					WHY?
15	☺	😍	😕	☹	😨	
16	☺	😍	😕	☹	😨	
17	☺	😍	😕	☹	😨	
18	☺	😍	😕	☹	😨	
19	☺	😍	😕	☹	😨	
20	☺	😍	😕	☹	😨	
21	☺	😍	😕	☹	😨	

One pound at a time

Exercise Tracker — Day 15 - 21

Day 15	Day 16	Day 17
Cardio ◯ Weights ◯	Cardio ◯ Weights ◯	Cardio ◯ Weights ◯

Day 18	Day 19	Day 20
Cardio ◯ Weights ◯	Cardio ◯ Weights ◯	Cardio ◯ Weights ◯

Day 21	Day	Calories Burned
	15	
	16	
	17	
	18	
	19	
Cardio ◯	20	
Weights ◯	21	

Day 15 Food Tracker

◎ **Daily Target**

Breakfast	Calories	Fat	Protein	Carbs	Fiber	Net Carbs
Total:						

Lunch	Calories	Fat	Protein	Carbs	Fiber	Net Carbs
Total:						

Dinner	Calories	Fat	Protein	Carbs	Fiber	Net Carbs
Total:						

Snacks	Calories	Fat	Protein	Carbs	Fiber	Net Carbs
Total:						

| **Daily Total** | | | | | | |

Ketosis: Y/N   Intermittent Fasting: From ____am/pm - To____am/pm

How'd I do?

Day 16 Food Tracker

Date: _____
MON TUE WED THU FRI SAT SUN

⌖ Daily Target						

Breakfast	Calories	Fat	Protein	Carbs	Fiber	Net Carbs
Total:						

Lunch	Calories	Fat	Protein	Carbs	Fiber	Net Carbs
Total:						

Dinner	Calories	Fat	Protein	Carbs	Fiber	Net Carbs
Total:						

Snacks	Calories	Fat	Protein	Carbs	Fiber	Net Carbs
Total:						

Daily Total						

Ketosis: Y/N   Intermittent Fasting: From _____am/pm - To_____am/pm

How'd I do?

Day 17 Food Tracker

🎯 Daily Target						

Breakfast	Calories	Fat	Protein	Carbs	Fiber	Net Carbs
Total:						

Lunch	Calories	Fat	Protein	Carbs	Fiber	Net Carbs
Total:						

Dinner	Calories	Fat	Protein	Carbs	Fiber	Net Carbs
Total:						

Snacks	Calories	Fat	Protein	Carbs	Fiber	Net Carbs
Total:						

Daily Total						

Ketosis: Y/N   Intermittent Fasting: From _____am/pm - To_____am/pm

How'd I do?

Day 18 Food Tracker

Date: _____
MON TUE WED THU FRI SAT SUN

⊕ Daily Target						

Breakfast	Calories	Fat	Protein	Carbs	Fiber	Net Carbs
Total:						

Lunch	Calories	Fat	Protein	Carbs	Fiber	Net Carbs
Total:						

Dinner	Calories	Fat	Protein	Carbs	Fiber	Net Carbs
Total:						

Snacks	Calories	Fat	Protein	Carbs	Fiber	Net Carbs
Total:						

Daily Total						

Ketosis: Y/N   Intermittent Fasting: From _____am/pm - To_____am/pm

How'd I do?

Day 19 Food Tracker

Date: _____

MON TUE WED THU FRI SAT SUN

🎯 Daily Target						

Breakfast	Calories	Fat	Protein	Carbs	Fiber	Net Carbs
Total:						

Lunch	Calories	Fat	Protein	Carbs	Fiber	Net Carbs
Total:						

Dinner	Calories	Fat	Protein	Carbs	Fiber	Net Carbs
Total:						

Snacks	Calories	Fat	Protein	Carbs	Fiber	Net Carbs
Total:						

Daily Total						

Ketosis: Y/N   Intermittent Fasting: From _____am/pm - To_____am/pm

How'd I do?

Day 20 Food Tracker

Date: _____
MON TUE WED THU FRI SAT SUN

⊕ Daily Target						
Breakfast	Calories	Fat	Protein	Carbs	Fiber	Net Carbs
Total:						
Lunch	Calories	Fat	Protein	Carbs	Fiber	Net Carbs
Total:						
Dinner	Calories	Fat	Protein	Carbs	Fiber	Net Carbs
Total:						
Snacks	Calories	Fat	Protein	Carbs	Fiber	Net Carbs
Total:						
Daily Total						

Ketosis: Y/N   Intermittent Fasting: From ____am/pm - To____am/pm

How'd I do?

Day 21 Food Tracker

Date: _____

MON TUE WED THU FRI SAT SUN

⊕ Daily Target						
Breakfast	Calories	Fat	Protein	Carbs	Fiber	Net Carbs
Total:						
Lunch	Calories	Fat	Protein	Carbs	Fiber	Net Carbs
Total:						
Dinner	Calories	Fat	Protein	Carbs	Fiber	Net Carbs
Total:						
Snacks	Calories	Fat	Protein	Carbs	Fiber	Net Carbs
Total:						
Daily Total						

Ketosis: Y/N   Intermittent Fasting: From _____am/pm - To_____am/pm

How'd I do?

Day 21
Ending Weight
and
Measurements

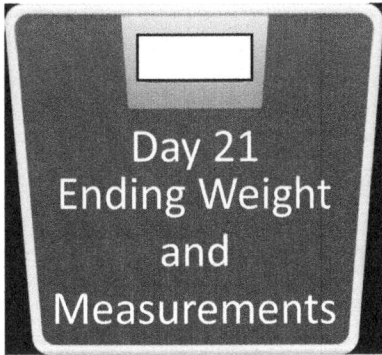

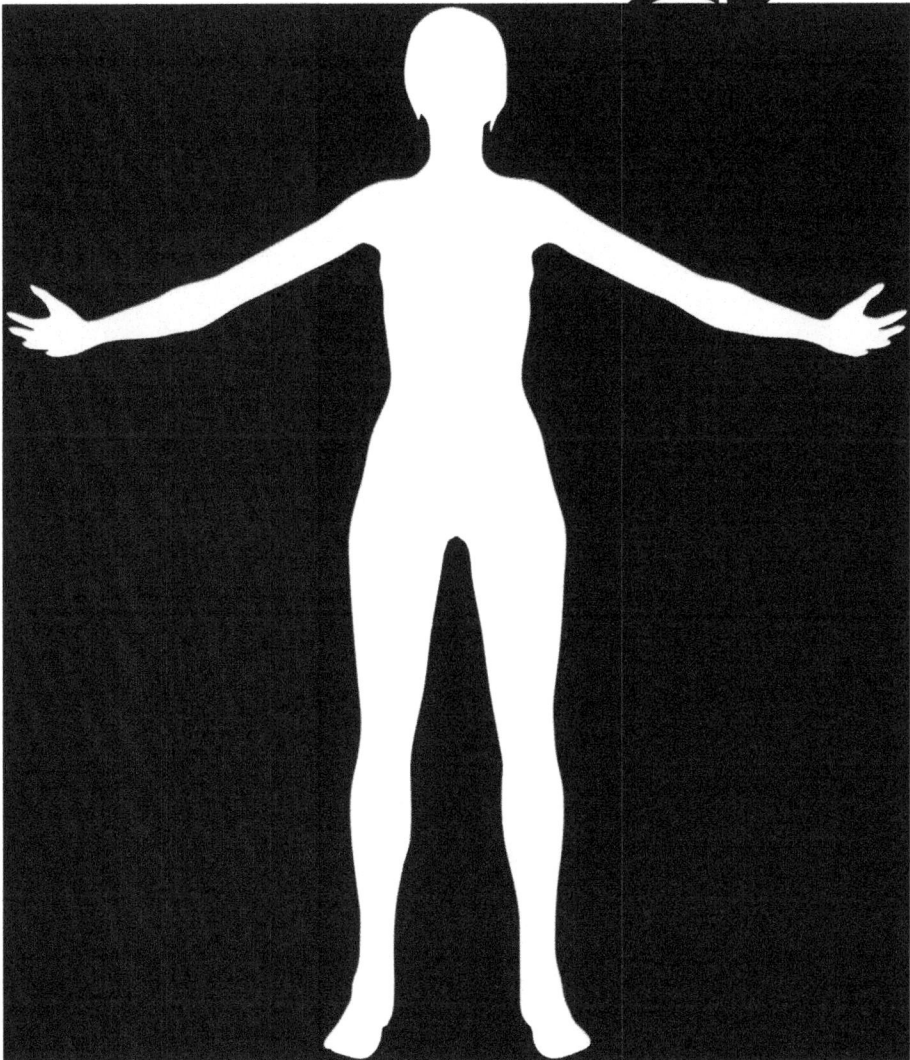

Strive for progress, not perfection

Weight +/- _____

Total Weight +/- _____

After 21 Days

4"x6"

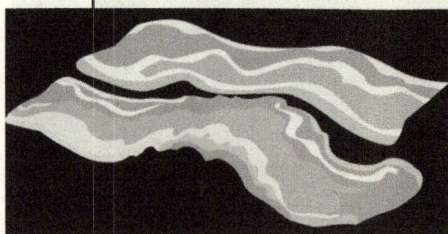

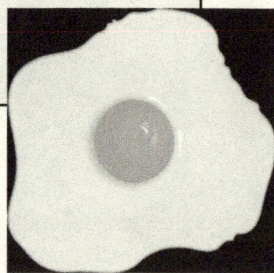

Questions To Ask Yourself

Will I continue with this way of eating? Why or why not?

_____

_____

_____

_____

Can I do this alone or do I need more support?

_____

_____

_____

Even if I reach my goal I will stick to Keto. True or False?

_____

_____

_____

I would recommend the Keto lifestyle to friends & family?

_____

_____

_____

I Can
&
I Did!

Keto

Recipes

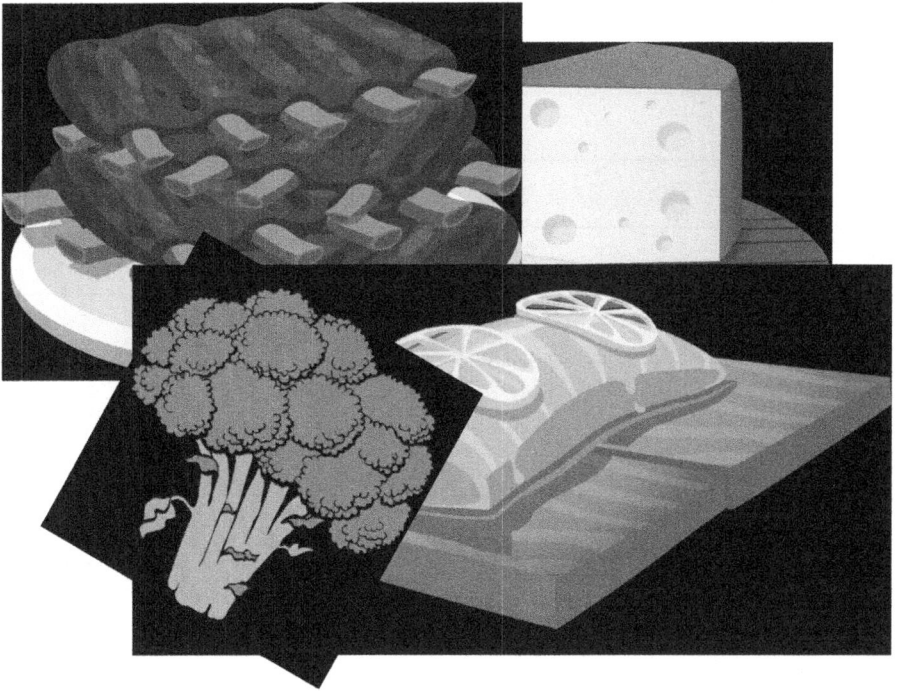

Recipe: _____

Prep Time [   ] Cook Time [   ] Servings [   ] Difficulty [   ]

Ingredients

_____

_____

_____

_____

_____

_____

_____

Directions

_____

_____

_____

_____

_____

_____

_____

_____

_____

_____

_____

Protein [   ] Fat [   ] Carbs [   ] Fiber [   ] Calories [   ]

Recipe: _____

Prep Time [   ] Cook Time [   ] Servings [   ] Difficulty [   ]

Ingredients

_____

_____

_____

_____

_____

_____

_____

_____

Directions

_____

_____

_____

_____

_____

_____

_____

_____

_____

_____

_____

_____

Protein [   ] Fat [   ] Carbs [   ] Fiber [   ] Calories [   ]

Recipe: _____

Prep Time [   ] Cook Time [   ] Servings [   ] Difficulty [   ]

Ingredients

_____

_____

_____

_____

_____

_____

_____

Directions

_____

_____

_____

_____

_____

_____

_____

_____

_____

_____

_____

Protein [   ] Fat [   ] Carbs [   ] Fiber [   ] Calories [   ]

Recipe: ───────────────

Prep Time [   ] Cook Time [   ] Servings [   ] Difficulty [   ]

Ingredients

_____

_____

_____

_____

_____

_____

Directions

_____

_____

_____

_____

_____

_____

_____

_____

_____

_____

Protein [   ] Fat [   ] Carbs [   ] Fiber [   ] Calories [   ]

Recipe: _____

Prep Time [   ] Cook Time [   ] Servings [   ] Difficulty [   ]

Ingredients

_____

_____

_____

_____

_____

_____

Directions

_____

_____

_____

_____

_____

_____

_____

_____

_____

_____

_____

Protein [   ] Fat [   ] Carbs [   ] Fiber [   ] Calories [   ]

Recipe: ——————————————

Prep Time [   ] Cook Time [   ] Servings [   ] Difficulty [   ]

Ingredients

_____

_____

_____

_____

_____

_____

_____

Directions

_____

_____

_____

_____

_____

_____

_____

_____

_____

_____

_____

Protein [   ] Fat [   ] Carbs [   ] Fiber [   ] Calories [   ]

Recipe: _____

Prep Time [   ] Cook Time [   ] Servings [   ] Difficulty [   ]

Ingredients

_____

_____

_____

_____

_____

_____

Directions

_____

_____

_____

_____

_____

_____

_____

_____

_____

_____

Protein [   ] Fat [   ] Carbs [   ] Fiber [   ] Calories [   ]

Recipe: _____

Prep Time [   ] Cook Time [   ] Servings [   ] Difficulty [   ]

Ingredients

_____

_____

_____

_____

_____

_____

_____

Directions

_____

_____

_____

_____

_____

_____

_____

_____

_____

_____

_____

_____

Protein [   ] Fat [   ] Carbs [   ] Fiber [   ] Calories [   ]

Recipe: _____

Prep Time [   ] Cook Time [   ] Servings [   ] Difficulty [   ]

Ingredients

_____

_____

_____

_____

_____

_____

_____

Directions

_____

_____

_____

_____

_____

_____

_____

_____

_____

_____

_____

Protein [   ] Fat [   ] Carbs [   ] Fiber [   ] Calories [   ]

Recipe: _____

Prep Time [   ] Cook Time [   ] Servings [   ] Difficulty [   ]

Ingredients

_____

_____

_____

_____

_____

_____

_____

Directions

_____

_____

_____

_____

_____

_____

_____

_____

_____

_____

_____

Protein [   ] Fat [   ] Carbs [   ] Fiber [   ] Calories [   ]

Recipe: _____

Prep Time [   ] Cook Time [   ] Servings [   ] Difficulty [   ]

Ingredients

_____

_____

_____

_____

_____

_____

Directions

_____

_____

_____

_____

_____

_____

_____

_____

_____

_____

Protein [   ] Fat [   ] Carbs [   ] Fiber [   ] Calories [   ]

Recipe: _____

Prep Time [　　] Cook Time [　　] Servings [　　] Difficulty [　　]

Ingredients

_____

_____

_____

_____

_____

_____

_____

Directions

_____

_____

_____

_____

_____

_____

_____

_____

_____

_____

_____

Protein [　　] Fat [　　] Carbs [　　] Fiber [　　] Calories [　　]

Recipe: ───────────────

Prep Time [   ] Cook Time [   ] Servings [   ] Difficulty [   ]

Ingredients

_____

_____

_____

_____

_____

_____

_____

Directions

_____

_____

_____

_____

_____

_____

_____

_____

_____

_____

_____

Protein [   ] Fat [   ] Carbs [   ] Fiber [   ] Calories [   ]

Recipe: ───────────────

Prep Time [   ] Cook Time [   ] Servings [   ] Difficulty [   ]

Ingredients

_____

_____

_____

_____

_____

_____

_____

Directions

_____

_____

_____

_____

_____

_____

_____

_____

_____

_____

_____

_____

Protein [   ] Fat [   ] Carbs [   ] Fiber [   ] Calories [   ]

Recipe: _____

Prep Time [   ] Cook Time [   ] Servings [   ] Difficulty [   ]

Ingredients

_____

_____

_____

_____

_____

_____

_____

Directions

_____

_____

_____

_____

_____

_____

_____

_____

_____

_____

_____

Protein [   ] Fat [   ] Carbs [   ] Fiber [   ] Calories [   ]

Recipe: _____

Prep Time [   ] Cook Time [   ] Servings [   ] Difficulty [   ]

Ingredients

_____

_____

_____

_____

_____

_____

_____

Directions

_____

_____

_____

_____

_____

_____

_____

_____

_____

_____

_____

Protein [   ] Fat [   ] Carbs [   ] Fiber [   ] Calories [   ]

Recipe: _____

Prep Time [   ] Cook Time [   ] Servings [   ] Difficulty [   ]

Ingredients

_____

_____

_____

_____

_____

_____

Directions

_____

_____

_____

_____

_____

_____

_____

_____

_____

_____

Protein [   ] Fat [   ] Carbs [   ] Fiber [   ] Calories [   ]

Recipe: _____

Prep Time [   ] Cook Time [   ] Servings [   ] Difficulty [   ]

Ingredients

_____

_____

_____

_____

_____

_____

_____

Directions

_____

_____

_____

_____

_____

_____

_____

_____

_____

_____

_____

Protein [   ] Fat [   ] Carbs [   ] Fiber [   ] Calories [   ]

Recipe: _____

Prep Time [   ] Cook Time [   ] Servings [   ] Difficulty [   ]

Ingredients

_____

_____

_____

_____

_____

_____

_____

Directions

_____

_____

_____

_____

_____

_____

_____

_____

_____

_____

Protein [   ] Fat [   ] Carbs [   ] Fiber [   ] Calories [   ]

Recipe: _____

Prep Time [   ] Cook Time [   ] Servings [   ] Difficulty [   ]

Ingredients

_____

_____

_____

_____

_____

_____

_____

Directions

_____

_____

_____

_____

_____

_____

_____

_____

_____

_____

_____

Protein [   ] Fat [   ] Carbs [   ] Fiber [   ] Calories [   ]

Recipe: _____

Prep Time [   ] Cook Time [   ] Servings [   ] Difficulty [   ]

Ingredients

_____

_____

_____

_____

_____

_____

Directions

_____

_____

_____

_____

_____

_____

_____

_____

_____

_____

_____

Protein [   ] Fat [   ] Carbs [   ] Fiber [   ] Calories [   ]

Recipe: ———————————

Prep Time [   ] Cook Time [   ] Servings [   ] Difficulty [   ]

Ingredients

_____

_____

_____

_____

_____

_____

Directions

_____

_____

_____

_____

_____

_____

_____

_____

_____

_____

Protein [   ] Fat [   ] Carbs [   ] Fiber [   ] Calories [   ]

Recipe: _____

Prep Time [   ] Cook Time [   ] Servings [   ] Difficulty [   ]

Ingredients

_____

_____

_____

_____

_____

_____

_____

Directions

_____

_____

_____

_____

_____

_____

_____

_____

_____

_____

Protein [   ] Fat [   ] Carbs [   ] Fiber [   ] Calories [   ]

Recipe: _____

Prep Time [   ] Cook Time [   ] Servings [   ] Difficulty [   ]

Ingredients

_____

_____

_____

_____

_____

_____

_____

Directions

_____

_____

_____

_____

_____

_____

_____

_____

_____

_____

_____

Protein [   ] Fat [   ] Carbs [   ] Fiber [   ] Calories [   ]

Recipe: _____

Prep Time [   ] Cook Time [   ] Servings [   ] Difficulty [   ]

Ingredients

_____

_____

_____

_____

_____

_____

_____

Directions

_____

_____

_____

_____

_____

_____

_____

_____

_____

_____

_____

_____

Protein [   ] Fat [   ] Carbs [   ] Fiber [   ] Calories [   ]

Recipe: _____

Prep Time [   ] Cook Time [   ] Servings [   ] Difficulty [   ]

Ingredients

_____

_____

_____

_____

_____

_____

_____

Directions

_____

_____

_____

_____

_____

_____

_____

_____

_____

_____

Protein [   ] Fat [   ] Carbs [   ] Fiber [   ] Calories [   ]

Recipe: _____

Prep Time [   ] Cook Time [   ] Servings [   ] Difficulty [   ]

Ingredients

_____

_____

_____

_____

_____

_____

_____

Directions

_____

_____

_____

_____

_____

_____

_____

_____

_____

_____

_____

Protein [   ] Fat [   ] Carbs [   ] Fiber [   ] Calories [   ]

Recipe: ————————————

Prep Time [   ] Cook Time [   ] Servings [   ] Difficulty [   ]

Ingredients

_____

_____

_____

_____

_____

_____

_____

Directions

_____

_____

_____

_____

_____

_____

_____

_____

_____

_____

_____

Protein [   ] Fat [   ] Carbs [   ] Fiber [   ] Calories [   ]

Recipe: _____

Prep Time [   ] Cook Time [   ] Servings [   ] Difficulty [   ]

Ingredients

_____

_____

_____

_____

_____

_____

Directions

_____

_____

_____

_____

_____

_____

_____

_____

_____

_____

Protein [   ] Fat [   ] Carbs [   ] Fiber [   ] Calories [   ]

Recipe: ————————————

Prep Time [   ] Cook Time [   ] Servings [   ] Difficulty [   ]

Ingredients

_____

_____

_____

_____

_____

_____

_____

Directions

_____

_____

_____

_____

_____

_____

_____

_____

_____

_____

Protein [   ] Fat [   ] Carbs [   ] Fiber [   ] Calories [   ]

Recipe: _____

Prep Time [   ] Cook Time [   ] Servings [   ] Difficulty [   ]

Ingredients

_____

_____

_____

_____

_____

_____

_____

Directions

_____

_____

_____

_____

_____

_____

_____

_____

_____

_____

_____

Protein [   ] Fat [   ] Carbs [   ] Fiber [   ] Calories [   ]

Recipe: ─────────────

Prep Time [   ] Cook Time [   ] Servings [   ] Difficulty [   ]

Ingredients

_____

_____

_____

_____

_____

_____

_____

Directions

_____

_____

_____

_____

_____

_____

_____

_____

_____

_____

_____

Protein [   ] Fat [   ] Carbs [   ] Fiber [   ] Calories [   ]

Recipe: ───────────────

Prep Time [   ] Cook Time [   ] Servings [   ] Difficulty [   ]

Ingredients

_____

_____

_____

_____

_____

_____

_____

Directions

_____

_____

_____

_____

_____

_____

_____

_____

_____

_____

_____

Protein [   ] Fat [   ] Carbs [   ] Fiber [   ] Calories [   ]

Recipe: ⎯⎯⎯⎯⎯⎯⎯⎯⎯⎯

Prep Time [   ] Cook Time [   ] Servings [   ] Difficulty [   ]

Ingredients

_____

_____

_____

_____

_____

_____

_____

Directions

_____

_____

_____

_____

_____

_____

_____

_____

_____

_____

_____

Protein [   ] Fat [   ] Carbs [   ] Fiber [   ] Calories [   ]

Recipe: _____

Prep Time [   ] Cook Time [   ] Servings [   ] Difficulty [   ]

Ingredients

_____

_____

_____

_____

_____

_____

Directions

_____

_____

_____

_____

_____

_____

_____

_____

_____

_____

_____

Protein [   ] Fat [   ] Carbs [   ] Fiber [   ] Calories [   ]

Recipe: _____

Prep Time [   ] Cook Time [   ] Servings [   ] Difficulty [   ]

Ingredients

_____

_____

_____

_____

_____

_____

_____

Directions

_____

_____

_____

_____

_____

_____

_____

_____

_____

_____

Protein [   ] Fat [   ] Carbs [   ] Fiber [   ] Calories [   ]

Recipe: _____

Prep Time [   ] Cook Time [   ] Servings [   ] Difficulty [   ]

Ingredients

_____

_____

_____

_____

_____

_____

Directions

_____

_____

_____

_____

_____

_____

_____

_____

_____

_____

_____

Protein [   ] Fat [   ] Carbs [   ] Fiber [   ] Calories [   ]

Recipe: ———————————

Prep Time [   ] Cook Time [   ] Servings [   ] Difficulty [   ]

Ingredients

_____

_____

_____

_____

_____

_____

_____

Directions

_____

_____

_____

_____

_____

_____

_____

_____

_____

_____

_____

Protein [   ] Fat [   ] Carbs [   ] Fiber [   ] Calories [   ]

Recipe: _____

Prep Time [   ] Cook Time [   ] Servings [   ] Difficulty [   ]

Ingredients

_____

_____

_____

_____

_____

_____

Directions

_____

_____

_____

_____

_____

_____

_____

_____

_____

_____

_____

Protein [   ] Fat [   ] Carbs [   ] Fiber [   ] Calories [   ]

Recipe: _____

Prep Time [   ] Cook Time [   ] Servings [   ] Difficulty [   ]

Ingredients

_____

_____

_____

_____

_____

_____

_____

Directions

_____

_____

_____

_____

_____

_____

_____

_____

_____

_____

_____

Protein [   ] Fat [   ] Carbs [   ] Fiber [   ] Calories [   ]

Published by:

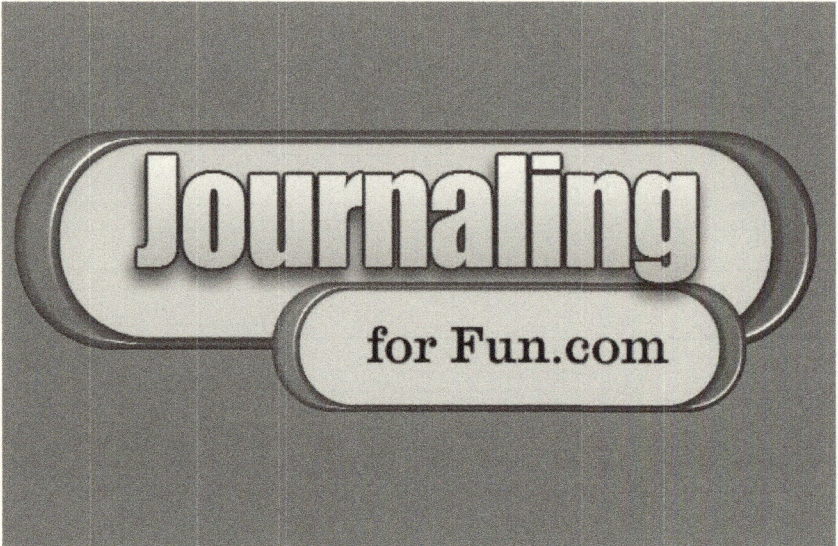

https://journalingforfun.com

Ron Kness

San Tan Valley, AZ

United States of America

Made in the USA
Las Vegas, NV
28 September 2022